Table of Contents

INTRODUCTION 1

CHAPTER 1 5
   WHAT IS STRESS?

CHAPTER 2 8
   WHO EXPERIENCES STRESS?

CHAPTER 3 12
   WHAT CAUSES STRESS?

CHAPTER 4 17
   WHAT ARE PHYSICAL SYMPTOMS OF STRESS?

CHAPTER 5 21
   HOW STRESS AFFECTS YOUR HEALTH AND WELL BEING

CHAPTER 6 25
   BREAKTHROUGH WAYS TO MANAGE AND REDUCE STRESS

CHAPTER 7 30
   BOX BREATHING – EXHALING ANXIETY

CHAPTER 8 35
   EXERCISE REGULARLY TO MANAGE STRESS BETTER.

CHAPTER 9 39
   REMOVING AND REDUCING KNOWN CAUSES OF STRESS

CHAPTER 10 43
   REDUCING OTHER POSSIBLE STRESSORS IN OUR LIVES

CHAPTER 11 47
  WAYS TO ELIMINATE STRESS

CHAPTER 12 68
  DEEP BREATHING FOR ANXIETY AND STRESS MANAGEMENT

CHAPTER 13 71
  MINDFULNESS TO MANAGE ANXIETY AND STRESS

CHAPTER 14 74
  LIVING WELL AT ANY AGE

CHAPTER 15 79
  HOW CAN WE DIFFUSE A STRESSFUL MOMENT OR PANIC ATTACK?

CHAPTER 16 88
  BENEFITS OF MEDITATION FOR NATURAL STRESS RELIEF

CLOSING 92

INTRODUCTION

In today's world, people are experiencing stress as a more normal part of their everyday lives. Throughout our day-to-day grind, we all need to find techniques to reduce and manage this stress and anxiety in order to keep ourselves and our friends and families healthier and happier.

Too much stress can affect our health, our relationships, our overall sense of self, and is something we should be aware of and take seriously. And it doesn't matter who you are, where you live, or even your age. We all have this one thing in common that can make our health and well being deteriorate, and we deal with it on a daily basis. And my goal is to help you help yourself or your loved ones such as a spouse, partner, friend or even your children, to better deal with this stress and recognize triggers so that they can feel more empowered to face whatever may come their way.

I have worked in private business, the medical field and in public education teaching high school students and spend a lot of time with elementary age children as a scout leader and mentor, and 'stress' does not belong to only adults. I have seen children of all ages affected by the stress in their lives. For adults and children, young and old, I have taught a technique that I will share with you that you can use, or share with your loved ones, to help manage and tackle the stress in their lives. By empowering our children with positive tools to deal with adversity in their lives we are setting them up for success later in life, not just to be successful academically or professionally but also successful in maintaining their overall health and well being.

Research has revealed that if people take time out to eliminate and manage their own stress levels, they can feel much better not only in the short-term but they also have the potential to benefit in the long-term with more positive outcomes for their overall health.

Of course, reducing stress and anxiety is easier said than done and in many cases just knowing how to reduce your stress and anxiety can be difficult in itself. My goal is to show you a way to take just a few minutes a day, so that you can begin lowering your stress and anxiety levels, and start to living a happier and healthier life.

You will discover the effects and the different causes. You are going to learn positive ways to cope with this problem by changing what we eat, and including physical activities into your life.

I think everyone at one time in their life have had to deal with some type of emotional problem that has taken a toll physically. Some of the things that can happen as a direct result would be a heart attack and high blood pressure. If you already have a disease or chronic condition, the strain could have effects such as depression or autoimmune disease.

Think about the times when you become strained and what the cause could have been. Perhaps you have financial or relationship troubles, or you face huge responsibilities at work that are a bit too much for you. If any of those hit home, then you have targeted the main issue. Start a journal where you mainly write when you feel overwhelmed or anxiety.

Everyone has automatic coping mechanisms like drinking too much liquor, or smoking. If you want to be honest with yourself, then you know this is not healthy in the least for the body.

However there are other things you can do which will affect everybody in a good way. We will go over those in a moment. You want to make healthy choices as opposed to harming your body further.

If you can make yourself relax, then you will be halfway there. Make a habit of meditating, or deep breathing. If you add some type of exercise to your daily life, doctors say that this helps the body and reduces anxiety.

Whatever you choose to do, just make sure that you do it on a regular basis. When you feel like you're getting anxious then you know how to relieve those feelings right away.

Doing anything physical and continuing relaxation exercises will prove to be extremely helpful both mentally and for a healthy body. Choose to eat healthier foods, and dropping all of your bad habits is a good thing.

Not all stress is bad, it is part of our natural survival mechanisms, we need it to push us either to perform feats like athletes, or when prepping for a difficult task, but our modern lives trigger this physiological response more and more subjecting our bodies and minds to stress and stress hormones.

It is beneficial in small amounts, but not long-term, then it can lead to a host of ill affects; premature aging, weakened immune function, cognitive and mood changes, and may even having lasting changes to the genes in our own bodies that we pass on to our children.

But, It's how we deal with it, and cope with stress that can make all the difference. And if we can teach our children to better deal with stress in positive, easy to manage ways, they can hopefully be more self-sufficient and be better prepared for all of life's challenges even when we aren't right by their side.

This guide will assist you in recognizing the impact of stress in our everyday lives and effective ways to reduce its toll.

Let's get started.

1 • WHAT IS STRESS?

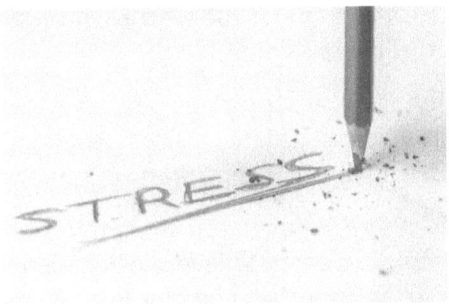

Stress refers to the strain from conflicts between our external environment and us, leading to emotional and physical pressure. It is not just a term that refers to someone in middle age toiling away in a cubicle from 9-5. In our fast paced world, it is impossible to live without stress, whether you are a student or a working adult.

There is both positive and negative stress, depending on each individual's unique perception of the tension between the two forces. Not all stress is bad. For example, positive stress, also known as eustress, can help an individual to function at optimal effectiveness and efficiency.

Hence, it is evident that some form of positive stress can add more color and vibrancy to our lives. The presence of a deadline, for example, can push us to make the most of our time and produce greater efficiency. Or an athlete that uses his or her stress response to push themselves to make the extraordinary happen.

It is important to keep this in mind, as stress management refers to using stress to our advantage, and not on eradicating the presence of stress in our lives.

On the other hand, negative stress can result in mental and physical strain. The individual will experience symptoms such as tensions, headaches, irritability and in extreme cases, heart palpitations.

Hence, whilst some stress may be seen as a motivating force, it is important to manage stress levels so that it does not have an adverse impact on your health and relationships.

Part of managing your stress levels include learning about how stress can affect you emotionally and physically, as well as how to identify if you are performing at your optimal stress level (OSL) or if you are experiencing negative stress.

This knowledge will help you to identify when you need to take a break, or perhaps seek professional help. It is also your first step towards developing techniques to managing your stress levels.

Modern day stresses can take the form of monetary needs, or emotional frictions. Competition at work and an increased workload can also cause greater levels of stress. How do you identify if you are suffering from excessive stress? How do you identify if your children seem to be suffering from excessive stress? Just as in the examples above, in their minds they can perceive the difficulties at home, they feel the pressure at school and within their peer groups and with the rise of social media their world may feel like it is caving in with the click of a screen or button.

Psychological symptoms commonly experienced include insomnia, headaches and an inability to focus. Physical symptoms take the form of heart palpitations, breathlessness, excessive sweating and stomachaches.

Common lifestyle stressors include performance, threat, and bereavement stressors, to name a few. Performance stressors are triggered when an individual is placed in a situation where he feels a need to excel. This could be during performance appraisals, lunch with the boss, or giving a speech.

Threat stressors are usually when the current situation poses a dangerous threat, such as an economic downturn, or from an accident. Lastly, bereavement stressors occur when there is a sense of loss such as the death of a loved one, or a prized possession.

Thus, there are various stressors, and even more varied methods and techniques of dealing with stress and turning it to our advantages. In order to do so, we must learn to tell when we have crossed the line from positive to negative stress.

2 • WHO EXPERIENCES STRESS?

Stress is something that affects everyone's lives. Stress is something that everybody endures on a fairly regular basis, but when it starts to impact negatively on your body and mind, it means you are not only stressed you may become distressed.

A lot of people don't realize how stress negatively impacts the body. In fact, stress has a bigger impact on our bodies than most of us care to acknowledge. Here are some facts about Stress and the effects on your body.

- 75-90% of all doctor visits are stress-related

Stress contributes to health problems such as heart disease, high blood pressure, obesity, and metabolic disorders such as diabetes.

- 43% of all adults have health problems related to stress

Stress also can cause or contribute to insomnia, changes in sex drive, mood and personality changes, substance abuse.

- Stress is known to cost American businesses more than $300 billion each year

The effects of stress lead to an increase in employee turnover, decreased productivity and job satisfaction and missed shifts, and higher insurance costs.

- More than 75% of adults report feeling stressed and more than a third of teenage students report the same.

These stats just target the adults, but children feel the effects of stress too. I've heard people ask, "What do kids have to be stressed about?" Really, they have much the same worries as adults, but they also illicit a stress response in their body over things adults might find trivial because we have the benefit or perspective of our years, we know the worlds not over just because we missed an assignment or so-and-so didn't wave back at school. And these are just the lighter examples, many children have to deal with stressors that would tax any adult, like, 'will we have food to eat tonight', 'are mom and dad going to have a job tomorrow', 'why do my parents always fight, are they going to divorce?', and a whole host of problems that we often overlook as affecting them because of their age or because they are peripherally affected.

Regardless of age or cause, constant exposure to stress keeps the body in 'fight-or-flight' mode, and stops being just an occasional occurrence and starts to become chronic, or persistent.

Chronic stress creeps up on you and gradually, as we fail to reduce or remove stressors from our life its effects will begin to manifest. At first, you may not even notice the symptoms of chronic stress at all, but if this stress is not managed, the symptoms can get worse and its effects may even be irreversible.

Stress can present and effect us in such a multitude of ways, here are seven ways we can all relate to, in which stress may manifest itself in your body are:

1. Anxiety. Those who are stressed are likely to deal with uncontrollable levels of anxiety. Anxiety and depression often go hand in hand, and this can cause

many different changes in the physiological functioning of the body.

2. Depression. When you are stressed out, it is very common for people to become depressed. There are only so many chemicals in the brain to help a person deal with stress, and when they are used up, they're used up. This can lead to a person becoming profoundly depressed in what seems like a relatively short period of time.

3. Diabetes. Type 2 diabetes is one of the fastest growing epidemics in the world and both mental and physical stress can cause rapid fluctuations in blood sugar levels. The long-term effects associated with this include heart disease, blindness, liver problems, kidney disease, and more.

4. Heart disease. Stress is very closely linked to heart attacks and death associated with cardiovascular disease. When stress is not managed, the body breaks down quickly and the heart is often profoundly impacted.

5. Obesity. We often cope with stress by consuming unhealthy, fattening foods. Plus, stress prohibits the control of necessary chemicals that are needed to break down fat, which can lead to obesity.

6. Sexual dysfunction. Stress is one of the most common reasons associated with impotence in men and lost libido in men and women.

7. Hair loss and premature greying. We often tease our friends and family when they begin to lose hair, but this can be a symptom of unmanaged stress. If your hair is falling out prematurely don't blame genetics, look

closely at how you are dealing with the stress in your life and see if there are things you can do to control it more effectively. And sure, Steve Martin and Anderson Cooper can rock a silver mane, but stress can be a factor that accelerates the ageing process that is visually evident as silvery streaks sometimes showing even in teens!

This is by no means an all-inclusive list of how stress affects your body and health. You may also suffer from hyperthyroidism, obsessive-compulsive disorder, tooth and gum disease, ulcers, and even cancer. Stress is serious stuff. This is all the more reason to start actively managing your stress today.

If your stress seems overwhelming, start trying to change things by adapting small strategies to combat your stress. Every little positive thing you do can lead to a big change.

3 • WHAT CAUSES STRESS?

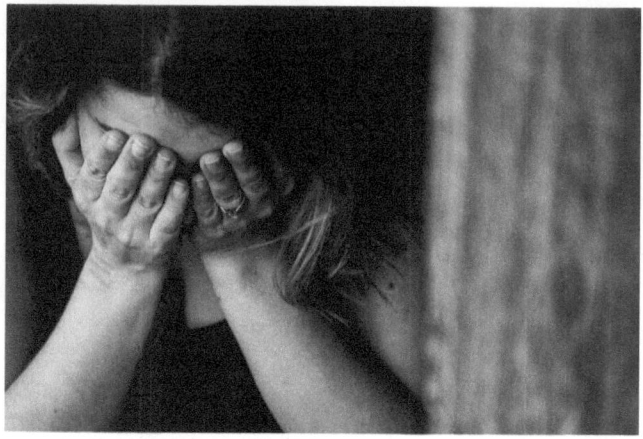

When it comes to stress, it must be said that in our modern world this is definitely a huge problem. Just as much as all of our innovations have helped us to be able to survive life on this planet more easily, it turns out that they are also what causes stress for us.

As much as our cars can take us from place to place so that travel is not arduous days of work, the cars also add pollution to the air we breathe, but that is not the only pollution they add. In fact, noise pollution is yet another side effect of our vehicles.

While it may seem a small price to pay for convenient travel, it has been shown that the finely tuned human auditory system is stressed by the noise from vehicles which most us can hear, even inside our homes. This is what causes stress on a small scale, but cars are clearly not the only culprits.

And when might that noise or the exhaust really start to set us off? When we are stuck in gridlock! We all need to get places and weather we ware behind the wheel or just a passenger, I think we can all agree that the feeling of not moving while time speeds on and we get further and further away from being to our destination on time is a huge stressor, and for many of us it is a twice daily ritual to sit and fume in our four wheeled prisons.

The situation is far more intricate than this. It has been shown, for example, that too much reading or TV viewing leads to eye strain. This kind of stress, while different, is equally tough on our nervous system and we get it in the name of being able to transfer knowledge more easily.

If TV is bad what about the glowing screens that seem to be attached to ours and our childrens hands. In an ideal world these miracles of technology should bring us closer together as we can connect to just about anyone, anywhere, at any time, but really think about how anxious we become if the 'wrong' name shows on the caller id or as a notification. Or how personally we feel assaulted by a strangers views on a post on social media, when we can spend less energy just setting the device down we invest so much energy and time into getting worked up and combatting some ethereal wrong in 140 characters or less.

To be clear, what causes stress is generally from outside of ourselves. Stress is a very natural function of the human body, a warning to us. If we heard a loud sound and experienced no stress from that, this could be deadly.

Millions of years of human evolution have given us the instinct to respond to sights, sounds and plenty of other sensory data that could save our lives. This is natural, but what is tough for us is when we cannot release the stress because the sensory data is not something we need to respond to.

Modern life.

But in our modern lives, these conveniences turn into stressors that our body responds to in the same way our ancient ancestors' bodies did when they were staring down some savage predator. Our physiology reacts gets us ready for fight or flight, even if it's just a text, tweet, or inconsiderate driver.

We all deal with stress every day.

Family Life

Our families can be a source of great joy, strength, and support; they can also be a source of a great deal of stress.

Raising children, and doing everything you can to make sure they are happy, healthy, and well cared for, can be pretty stressful. If you have several children, just keeping all of their individual schedules straight can be a major source of stress.

Relationship problems (like conflicts with your spouse, or divorce proceedings) can make the other stresses in your life seem even worse.

Work

Work is a pretty big source of stress. Working long hours, and dealing with a heavy workload, can leave little time for fun in your life.

Another source of stress is an unpleasant work environment. This can mean anything from a verbally abusive boss, to feuding coworkers, to a fellow employee who is making unwanted romantic advances towards you.

If you find yourself tensing up or feeling depressed before you even get to work in the morning that is a pretty clear indication that your job is a major source of stress in your life.

Finances

Financial problems are a major source of stress, not just on individuals, but on relationships as well. Many divorced and divorcing couples will cite financial problems as one of the major causes of their split. Constant worry about credit card debt, or the high cost of living, can make it hard for some to relax and enjoy life.

Image Issues

It almost seems like no one is happy with the way they look. Even many super models claim that there is at least one thing about their bodies that they hate.

Many people spend a great deal of their time and energy worrying about how they look and how much they weight. And they spend billions of dollars a year on cosmetic surgery, weight loss programs, and fad diets, trying to make themselves look the way they think they should.

The Wrong Ways to Deal With Stress

Considering how much stress we have to deal with every day, finding ways to deal with that stress is crucial. But the methods some use to deal with stress only make things worse. Some people turn to alcohol or other substances to relax and de-stress. But, when this use gets out of control, it creates bigger problems and more stress in your life and in the lives of your loved ones.

Some people find food comforting. When they're eating their favorite meal or snack, their problems seem to fade away for a while. However, relying on food too much can lead to weight gain, and weight is a major source of stress for many people.

No matter the substance; food, alcohol, or illicit, they will not take away the stress, they will not help the body, they will only do the opposite. They can exacerbate the problems and issues you already are combating and are not the best tool in your tool box.

You already are equipped with everything you need, and if you are reading to help a loved one, so are they. We all have to deal with stress and if you give me a little more of your time, my goal will be to help you breathe easier, and maybe lift some of the weight of this modern life off your shoulders.

4 • WHAT ARE PHYSICAL SYMPTOMS OF STRESS?

Most people are familiar with the feelings of discomfort, anxiety, depressed states and overall uneasiness that stress can cause. But in the words of the band Boston, "It's more than a feeling", of course I don't think those guys were crooning about stress, right? Stress not only affects the way we feel it has a real effect on our physical well-being. These effects can be simple as a blush in the cheeks or more severe like losing your hair. Even more worrisome, current scientific studies are looking at the connections between chronic stress and serious diseases and even higher incidences of cancers. The following are a few just a few examples of some of the ways stress can take a toll on your body.

Headaches

Stress headaches may sound like just a generic label if we can't find some other cause but many people suffering from chronic stress suffer also from chronic headaches. There are many causes such as clenching ones teeth when anxious or upset. Sometimes we don't even realize we are clenching or grinding our teeth because of stress, some even stress grind in their sleep. The pressure of clenching can cause discomfort, tension and inflammation in the jaw and facial muscles and may cause referred pain in the head and face that can lead to one form of stress related headache.

This pain or tension is not always localized to the face and head alone, for some people their tension headaches can start from tension carried in their necks, which too can drive these headaches.

Other stress headaches can be caused by the high levels of stress and anxiety affecting sleep patterns-headaches are a byproduct when we get less sleep.

Cardiovascular Disease

The longer and more frequent our body is under stress and the natural "fight-or-flight" response, the more time our body is flooded with stress hormones. We need those hormones, such as epinephrine, for acute or sudden stress to ensure survival in life or death situations. They speed up the heart and lungs and alter our blood pressure and kick us into high gear. But when our bodies are subjected to chronic stresses day after day those hormones start to wear out these vital organs and the network of blood vessels that carry our precious blood throughout the body. The prolonged exposure to stress can lead to increased blood pressure or hyper tension which can affect your bloods clotting, and when blood clotting is affected heart attack risk increases. The increased pressure on blood vessels can also lead to other vascular conditions including aneurisms, or burst vessels, which is extremely dangers and most of the times fatal because when a blood vessel such as an artery carrying blood from the heart bursts, you will bleed out before medical care can be received.

Weight Changes

I'm sure if you're like me you'd like to lose a pound or two, or twenty, but at what cost? Stress can have the effect of altering a person's physique moving the needle wither direction on the scale. Some people can't keep down food or have frequent diarrhea because of their stress and become nearly malnourished and lose weight.

Some may not have an appetite due to nausea from the way the stress hormones affect their stomachs.

While others use food to cope with their stress and anxieties and satiate their demons with calories, it could be comfort foods that reduce the stress or anxious binge eating. The increased caloric intake coupled with cortisol, the other stress hormone secreted from our adrenal gland can lea to increased fat conversion and storage in the body.

Body Aches & Chronic Muscle Pains

We often use the term mind over matter to describe a person's ability to power through a situation through sheer will, the mind is extremely powerful, unfortunately the negative thoughts can affect the body just as much as the positive. People who suffer from various chronic stresses often complain of generalized body aches or muscle pains and fatigue. The powerful stress hormones take a toll on the mind and body, their purpose is to accelerate the body for survival and self-preservation, but when our muscles are feeling their influence nearly every waking hour it literally wears them out, and just like wearing out your muscles in other ways, you feel pain. Stress is mentally and physically exhausting!

Changes to Sleep Cycle

Speaking of exhausting, I'm betting I'm not the only one who has been stressed or anxious and couldn't fall asleep at night. Many of us probably have laid in bed and felt as if we just couldn't turn our brains off, and every time we look at a clock and see the hours rapidly ticking by and our window to sleep shrinking and our anxiety and stress levels rising.

Chronic stress and the stress hormones our body produces can alter and affect our regular wake/sleep cycle and keep us from getting our best nights sleeps, it can lead to insomnia, and the lack of sleep takes an even further toll on our bodies.

For others, their sleep cycles are affected in the opposite direction, as the stress levels rise, so do their hours spent sleeping, this is hypersomnia, so they have troubles staying awake, or when awake feel sluggish, lethargic and fatigued.

5 • HOW STRESS AFFECTS HEALTH & WELL BEING

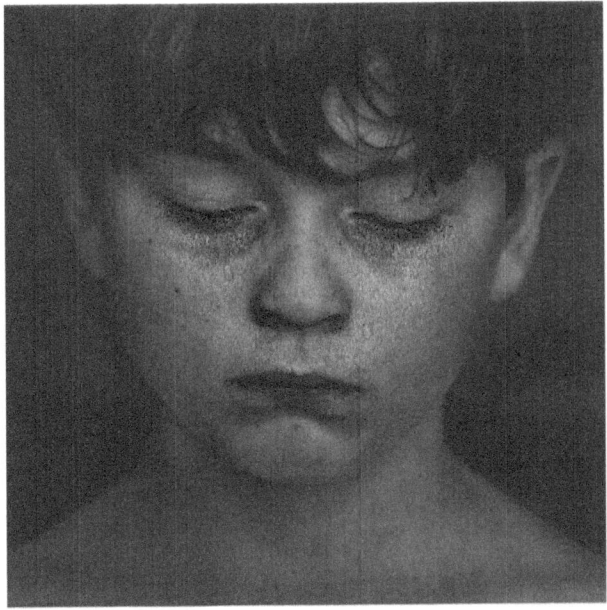

It's not uncommon for people to ask, "How does stress affect health?" We may hear stories about how stress can ruin you physically and mentally. Is there any truth to it?

The truth is that researchers are still trying to determine the exact effects of stress. Several studies show a tentative but strong connection between stress and certain health problems; some things are fairly certain though.

Studies show for example that at the most, 90% of complaints in clinics are due to stress with 43% of people suffering badly from stress. OSHA, the Occupational Safety and Health Administration, has stated that stress is a major work hazard.

The following pages ouline just some of the ways stress can affect your long-term health and wellness.

1. Stress may be responsible for certain heart ailments and conditions. The hormones produced during a state of stress increase blood pressure and heart rate. This increase will in turn put too much pressure on the arteries. This could harm them, cause them to thicken, and eventually lead to, or accelerate the onset of, heart disease.

2. Stress takes a major toll on your immune system; people under chronic stress tend to be more prone to colds and infections. This is because the hormone cortisol which is present in large amounts when under stress tends to hinder the work of the immune system.

3. Metabolic disorders and weight fluctuations, you'll may gain additional weight when under increased stress. This is due to the body's quick use of carbohydrate stores. This in turn could encourage you to eat more. On the flip side, those who are too busy to even eat could lose weight and consume all of their energy stores. That would leave them with nothing to draw energy and nutrients from.

4. You may have noticed that you may experience more stomach complaints when under stress. If you miss meals due to your preoccupation with stressful factors, then you could develop hyperacidity. Loose bowels are also a natural reaction to stress due to chemical reactions that cause the stomach to digest food improperly.

5. Your physical well being is not the only victim of your stress, your mental and psychological state is also in danger. Stress naturally produces and increases anxiety, worry and frustration. These could lead to the development of more serious psychological conditions such as depression, mood swings, and possibly more serious suicidal thoughts and ideations.

6. Stress can rob you of your sleep, a good night sleep is the body's way of recharging itself so you can face the next day with renewed energy. If you lose sleep, your body would not have been rested well enough. This naturally takes its toll on your daily performance. Your mind is taxed by the lack of sleep which only increases stress levels and, the rest of your body feels the pressure and suffers too since it has been in working mode from dusk till dawn.

7. Those who experience stress complain of a variety of other conditions. You may experience, headaches, body aches, rashes, gum problems, menstrual irregularities, hair loss and sexual problems. Stress affects and afflicts everyone in in differing ways because we are all different, not only in genetic make-up and anatomy, but also in how we handle and manage those stressors in our lives.

Suffice it to say that whatever your stress threshold is, it is best to keep your stress levels below that threshold over the long term. Monitor yourself for stress symptoms and be prepared to take action when they are detected.

Stress and anxiety are serious health issues that you cannot afford to ignore for long. The good news is that there are effective techniques for managing stress that you can use to avoid its negative health effects.

We are almost to the technique I want to share with you to deal with the stressors in your life, so how about a little stress relief practice to get us there.

In a moment I want you to just close your eyes and focus on your breathing. Nothing special except try to clear your thoughts of whatever may be weighing on you and just focus on the movement of air in your nose and out of your mouth.

Let's give that a try.

Maybe half a minute to a minute (or more, no rush I'll wait!)

So…close your eyes and breathe…

Feel a little better? Good!

Let's not stop now!

6 • BREAKTHROUGH WAYS TO MANAGE AND REDUCE STRESS

There have always only been twenty-four hours in a day and three hundred and sixtyfive days in a year, but it seems that people are trying to pack more into their per hour, minute and day than ever before. The more that is accomplished, the greater the level of future expectation becomes.

As demands on a person's time become more and more pronounced, the pressure to do escalates and the result is often stress, anxiety or depression. None of those three things are what anyone wants. However, of the three, stress and anxiety are the easiest to manage. Depression is a very serious medical condition and don't let anyone ever tell you or your loved one other wise.

Depression is a common mental health problem and is significantly different from mere unhappiness or sadness. Depression is related to changes in the levels of certain chemicals in the brain.

These changes can make the depression very difficult to break out of without treatment. It is clear that stress is usually not as acute as depression, and it is stress that will be discussed here.

Stress is the most common aliment or underlying cause of ill health, of our modern age. It has been found to be part of the cause of a host of conditions that we've talked about so far such as peptic ulcer disease, coronary heart disease, depression, autoimmune disease, hypertension, diabetes and even cancer.

And stress is so significant because it brings with it feelings of loss of control or lack of choice during particular situations. This lack of control makes people feel trapped, anxious and often helpless to affect change in their situation. Stress and its effects are also a major factor and driver in mental health, especially anxiety and depression.

Now that it is established exactly what stress is and how dangerous the more severe cases can be, the question becomes what can be done about it? First, develop "flexible control" in your life.

Know that you cannot control every detail of your life. Life is unpredictable and sometimes things just happen that are out of your control. Developing self-acceptance skills will assist in numerous ways. One of the main reasons is that this will prevent the negative consequences of low self-esteem and self-worth when we blame ourselves for things outside of our control.

Here are some sure-fire "flexible control" ideas to reduce stress levels in your life and make it a little more manageable, this will allow you to use the good and moderate stress levels in your life to warn you about things that you need to pay attention to. It's important to listen to your body and the alerts it gives you.

1. Short bursts of breathing, meditation, daydreaming, sitting with a cup of tea or even simply staring out the window will produce a calming effect and reduce stress.

2. Get up fifteen minutes earlier each morning. That gives you a little more time to eat something, run back

to get something you forgot, or enjoy a cup of coffee before heading out the door.

3. Write it down. Write down goals, errands, chores, due dates for projects and library books. In addition to a "To Do" list, keep a "Have Done" list too.
4. Do something special and totally unexpected on a whim.
5. Assume that others are doing the best they can and be willing to forgive when the situation arises. Learning to forgive others goes a long way in showing you how to forgive yourself.

These five points above are terrific way to start to reduce or eliminate certain stresses in your life; a couple additional things you can do:

Delegate new jobs. Say "no" to avoid additional responsibilities. Learn to ignore others' criticism. Walking and Jogging is another great way to reduce stress in your life and improve your overall health.

Another great way to reduce stress in your life is to take a vacation. These don't have to be long, expensive, extravagant affairs. They can be just staying in town with your family for the weekend or setting aside a day or two of 'me time'. Vacations are meant to be a way to escape from the usual grind and busy times and get a different perspective. Be careful though, don't try to do too much on your vacation and plan everything out.

If you do, that relaxing time you planned just becomes work. Keeping up with schedules and deadlines when you try to cram too much into your holiday never works. It will just lead to more stress, ironically the very thing you are trying to avoid. How many times have you said, "I need a weekend from my weekend!", I know it can't just be me!

Stress can also be reduced though simple breathing exercises that you can do wherever you are. These are what we will be focusing on as our primary tool that you can literally do anytime, anywhere, and at any age. In the next chapter we will look at the technique called 'Box Breathing' that has been shown to physiologically change the body by simply controlling your breathing.

Things like breathing and meditation help by refocusing your attention elsewhere for a brief period. Meditation and stress relief exercises restore the body to a calm state, helping it repair itself and prevent any damage. The physical effect of meditation on our bodies decreases our heart rate and slows breathing.

Not all stress can or should be avoided. Learning how to recognize when too many things are crowding into your life and being able to say no at appropriate times is one the best things that you can do for yourself and the people that you care about.

If you see someone whom you think is overstressed today, take them aside and warn them of the physical and emotional dangers of such a course. You can educate them about our breathing exercises, meditation and practicing mindfulness. Doing all these things will help you build up both psychological and physiological defenses against future stress.

This however is not a one-time fix. Be on guard against future increases in stress levels. Catching yourself experiencing these things early means that you are more in control of your own life. One key is maintaining a proper physical, spiritual, and emotional balance in your life.

Stress relief is not about escaping stress; it's about keeping everything in perspective. Meditation practices teach the basic skill of how to live in the present for fifteen to twenty minutes. But mindfulness skills teach you to live a more centered life, day in day out. Doing these things will help you not only be healthier but hopefully happier too.

7 • BOX BREATHING – EXHALING ANXIETY

I've talked frequently about controlling and managing stress with breathing; we can do this by just taking time to relax and catch our breath or give ourselves a moment to cool off. And if we want to combat the effects of chronic stress, we need something we can easily add to our daily routine. With this technique I will teach you is a way to do both, fight sudden and chronic stress, and physiologically alter your body. What do I mean by that? I mean you can change the way your body functions and start to affect to automatic autonomic processes that make up our stress response and normal feedback mechanisms in the body. It can calm the body and return it to a more normalized state and rhythm when things start getting hectic and chaotic. I want to teach you to breathe the stress out, to exhale your anxieties.

This technique is most commonly called box breathing, or square breathing, and is an easy yet powerful tool to help you manage your stress. This method of breathing to control anxiety and decrease stress was first popularized for its use by the U.S. Navy SEALs, you may have heard it called the Navy SEAL breathing technique or tactical breathing. But you don't have to be a member of our eite fighting forces to employ this fantastic tool, we can all master it. And if you are reading this because you want to help out your children, you're in luck, even 4 and 5-year olds can get the hang of it! No special equipment necessary, you can do it anytime, anywhere.

Let's get to breathing.

To get started and get practiced at the technique, I suggest finding a quiet place to start your first box breathing sessions. This will help limit distractions and help you focus on your breaths and the changes in you mind and body.

This technique is called box or square breathing because it has 4 basic steps, and it can be helpful as we clear our minds to visualize this box or square.

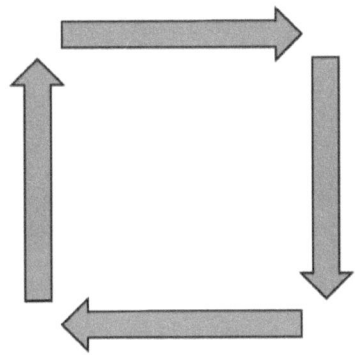

As we make our way around the sides of this box we will perform the technique.

Step 1 - Breathe in through your nose for three seconds.

Step 2 - Hold that breath for three seconds.

Step 3 - Exhale through your mouth for three seconds.

Step 4 – Hold for three seconds.

Repeath these steps for 10-15 cycles or 2-3 minutes.

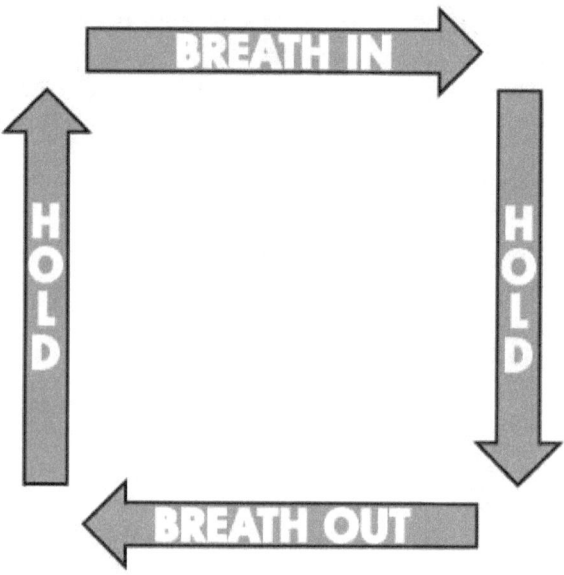

As you complete these repetitions you will begin to feel the release of tension and stress and you focus on your breathing. Not only will the slow inhale of oxygen make you feel better, but you will experience the release of stress as you exhale.

Once you get more practiced and comfortable with the technique you will want to increase your count used on your breaths, such as moving up to five seconds per step, and continuing the cycle for about 5 minutes per session.

And this is it. It is so simple, yet so very powerful. Anyone can do this, and it will make a world of difference for you, your family, and anyone else you share it with. You will begin to take charge of the negative things in your mind and those emotions and stresses that are causing you pain.

When you perform this box breathing technique, you will move your body into a calmer state. This is you affecting your physiology, or the functioning of your body. You will start to influence processes that are not necessarily voluntary and put yourself in a position to better manage your own well being.

You will slow your heart rate and lower your blood pressure by improving blood flow, not permanently, but you will have a new tool to call upon when you feel your heart start to race or the pressure rise.

You can clear your mind and increase focus and concentration using this technique. I often start class with a box breathing session to get my students in an improved state of mind for the lesson they are about to tackle. I've use this too with groups of cub scouts to help them settle from an activity and help them calm themselves down, so they can focus on our meetings.

If you or your loved ones ever feel that they can't fall to sleep at night because you feel like you 'just can't shut your brain off.' This is the perfect technique as you lay in bed; you will clear your mind, relax your body, and find yourself falling to sleep far easier and quicker than before.

If you already meditate or are getting in meditation or mindfulness practices to manage your stress, box breathing is a perfect partner to help clear your thoughts and set your focus and state of mind.

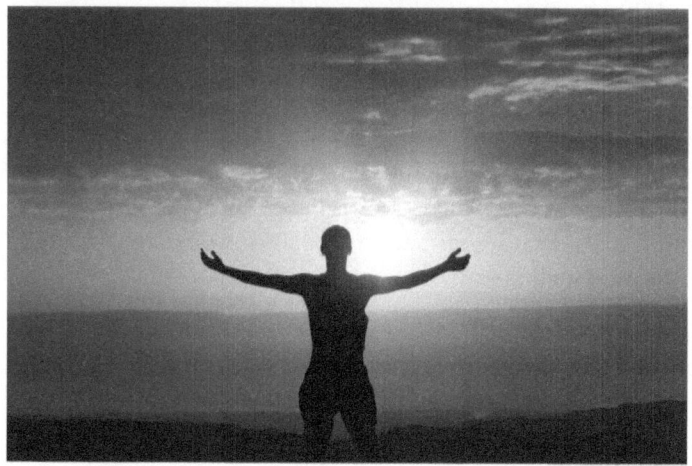

8 • EXERCISE REGULARLY TO MANAGE STRESS BETTER.

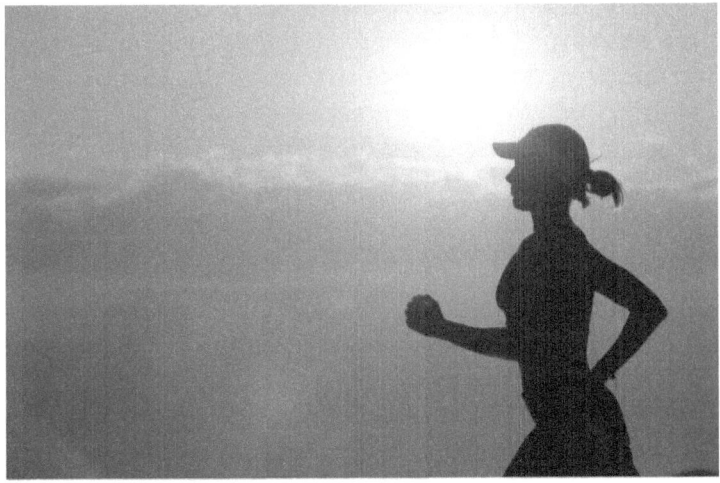

Managing Stress is as much a physical issue as it is a psychological concern. To boost the benefits of counseling, experts of stress management and therapists keep advising their clients to get busy in some type of exercise training program.

People who are suffering from extreme stress often complain of weakness, sluggishness and generalized malaise in going about daily work and may feel that they are unable to perform to their fullest.

So, you're determined to go through a stress management exercise program, how do you even begin? If you have not been active for a long time and have been leading a sedentary life, the best way to start is by walking.

It can become quite enjoyable for sure when you take pleasure in small things like noticing surroundings - the green plants around, the chirping of birds, the different types of buildings, the people around, etc. Walking daily is a great exercise and eventually not only will you start to feel better but you'll probably notice you are less stressed too. Walking is a great time to practice breathing and mindfulness techniques, you can perform your box breaths as you circle the block or cross the park. And when walking alone, this can be your own little get away in your busy day.

While starting on a stress management exercising program, keep in mind that exercise trains but too much of it can strain. This means that you should work at a comfortable pace and level. If you overburden yourself, or jump in too much too fast, there are chances that you will get more stressed than before and may give up or stop before you realize the benefits of exercise.

You should exercise at a level and frequency that you enjoy and become healthier rather than causing harm to yourself. Have fun while walking, running, or hitting the gym and enjoy every movement of your body without any strain.

You don't need to be a professional runner to achieve the beneficial effects of a stress management program. In fact, researchers have proven that any physical exercise of moderate nature 30-40 minutes daily gives many health benefits. By moderate, we mean exercises like cycling, gardening, brisk walking and performing household chores.

Since physical exercise requires good concentration, you will have no time to think about your problems. This will slowly help to rid you of the stress and anxieties that linger in your mind. This is a type of selective awareness. Strenuous exercise can provide even better results and benefits. To obtain cardiovascular benefits from strenuous exercises, the heart rate should be raised to 60%-80% level. Of course, check with your healthcare provider before beginning any new strenuous exercise regimine, everyone's health history is different.

For the desired results of the training program, you should exercise 20-30 minutes for 3-4 days every week. Since cardio respiratory endurance decreases after 48 hrs, you must ensure that you exercise at least three days in a week. You can schedule your exercise into your daily routine in a manner most comfortable to you and your schedule.

This way, you will approach it like a commitment that has to be kept and will be more than ready to exercise rather than finding excuses to exercise when you get time and putting it off continuously for a later date.

To assess and properly find out how your body is responding to specific types of exercises, learn to listen to the body. The following are some signs of over exhaustion that give you signals to cut down on your exercise routine.

- Muscle and joint Soreness

- Feeling of heavy in arms and legs

- Continuously feeling tired

- Inabilty to relax

- Bad appetite
- Under weight
- Problem such as Constipation and diarrhea
- Repeatedly getting injured

9 • REMOVING AND REDUCING KNOWN CAUSES OF STRESS

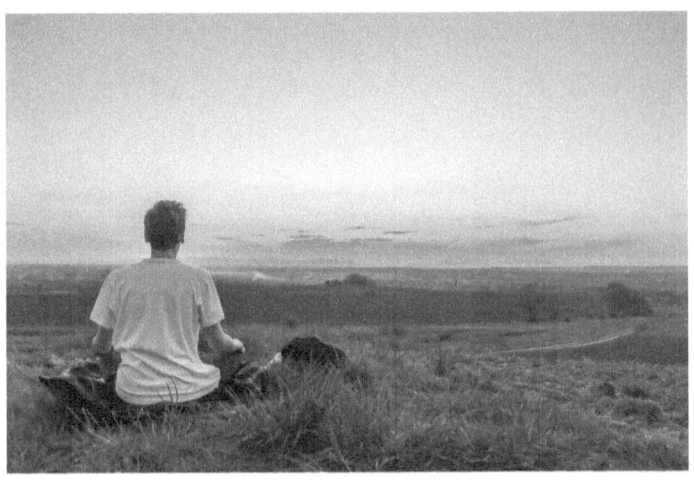

Meditation, relaxation and visualization are the standard recommendations for reducing stress, and they are all beneficial and useful to us in many ways, however, they are not so easy to put into use when stress strikes with its disruptive companions such as frustration, confusion, anxiety, and feeling overwhelmed, are in full attendance.

Here's something simple you can try to diffuse stress quickly and easily, anytime and anywhere.

1.   Rub your forehead with both hands in vertical lines from your eyebrows to your hairline for a few moments

2.   About an inch above each eyebrow you will find a bump - rest your fingertips there lightly and hold

3.   Take a deep breathe in and lighten the pressure of your fingertips until they are touching those points very softly

4.   Breathe deeply again and allow yourself to sink into how you are really feeling right now - focus clearly and specifically on the one thing that is mainly causing you stress, or anxiety

5.   Allow yourself to think the truth of the matter, hold the points and breathe and remain that way for a couple of minutes

6.   Concentrate on the area you are holding and feel for pulsations under your fingertips as the blood flow, previously diverted by stress, is restored to your forebrain. Now you can begin to think clearly again as you feel stress drain away and find yourself in control and able to choose how you wish to respond to what's at hand.

What many of us don't realise about stress is that although it is often triggered by our mental states and emotional responses, it is in fact a physiological occurrence. The body responds directly to every impression we feed it be it real or imagined; it makes no difference to the body.

If you tell it you are stressed it will respond immediately by sending the majority of the blood from your forebrain to your chest for faster breathing and the more efficient pumping of blood through your heart and to the muscles of your legs for whatever action they may need to take.

When you consider this automatic physical response it's easy to see why we don't always think well under stress. This simple technique tells your body to stand down and encourages the blood flow to return to the brain for clear thinking and decision-making.

Try this technique for:

1. Diffusing stress on the spot and stopping it from accumulating
2. Easing worries and helping with panic attacks
3. Regaining control of your resources and having access to your full capacity for dealing with any given situation.
4. Preventing the digestive disorders associated with stress developing. (Use this before eating to make sure that your digestive system is ready and willing to

receive the goodness from your food in a calm and efficient manner.)

5. Relaxing and clearing your mind before sleep
6. Inducing a feeling of calm from which you can then step deeper into a meditative or relaxed state

10 • REDUCING OTHER POSSIBLE STRESSORS IN OUR LIVES

As we've covered, long term stress is bad for us and can do irreparable harm as we age and even accelerate the process so let us look at some additional ways we can slow down the clock and reduce stress.

This chapter lays out a handful tweaks, habits and easy to manage lifestyle changes that we can all get behind, some may work for you some may not, it's always good to have plenty of tools at your disposal.

1. Breathing. As we've covered, and I can't stress enough (pun intended.) The more stressed, anxious, and hurried we become, the less we remember to take deep, full breaths. Your cells need that precious oxygen for energy and to properly metabolize and mobilize cellular waste. Your brain needs oxygen, just like it needs fuel, in order to work at optimum levels ensuring the best brain chemistry to help us reduce stress.

When you take shallow breaths, your body has to work harder to function normally. Take a few minutes out of your day to practice breathing deeply. Focus on the movement of the air in and out of the lungs, exhaling fully, holding your breath, and inhaling.

2. Get Active and Moving. Movement works your muscles, gets the blood flowing, it stimulates your nervous system, and encourages you to breathe more deeply, bringing in additional oxygen to the body. Studies

are showing that even short bursts of exercise such as a walk a day can be just as beneficial as hittitting the gym. Exercise has also been shown to help keep your brain sharp -so to maintain a clear, quick intellect, make sure you get out and move your body daily, even if it's just walking the dog around the block. Also beneficial are body-mind practices, such as meditation, yoga or qi gong. These excellent additions can help focus your attention on places you're holding stress and tension in your body, allowing you to consciously release them.

3. Declutter to destress! Reorganize your home, office, or personal space. Chaos breeds chaos, and a messy space can create mental clutter as well. If your home isn't a sanctuary, consider spending a Saturday doing a deep cleaning. It can also be thearapeatuic and cathartic to take your mind off the problems of the world around you.

And while you are doing some good for yourself, you can do some good for those in need. As you clear out clutter that you no longer need, donate it to a local Women's Shelter, Salvation Army or other charity that can get it to someone who needs it.

4. Use a relaxing fragrance to soothe your mind. Fragrance can deeply effect our psyche, it can conjure closely held memories and feelings and take you to a happy place. Scented candles or essential oil diffusers can easily be used in your home and sometimes office. Some people find Lavender essential oil to be soothing, Peppermint uplifting, and Rosemary can be energizing. I

personally am soothed by the smell of coffee, that's my happy place, but that does lead to my next point...

5. Cut back on caffeine. Okay, I know this is probably a tough one for most of us; I've been known for having a bit of an excessive coffee habit. With that in mind, if you feel yourself constantly jumpy, notice your hands are shaky, or you struggle with nervousness and anxiousness, consider limiting the coffee you drink. Switching to a different caffeine source can also do the trick. Green, or flavored tea are good options for some people.

6. Meditate. Ugh. You mean sit still and clear my mind of all thoughts? Yep, that's what I mean. When you're stressed out, the committee in your head gets louder and louder until you can't hear yourself think anymore. You may even forget what you think.

If sitting quietly sounds about as much fun to you as getting a root canal, try joining a meditation group. The accountability and community support can make the experience fun and relaxing instead of another arduous task to complete. For some, myself included, I prefer to practice walking meditation, I try to find time in the morning when it is quiet and unhurried, and get a meditative walk in. What if you are time crunched?

Try a meditation CD or youtube channel to help you drop into peace and tranquility.

7. Unplug. We're under constant assault of messages, advertisements headlines, alerts, buzzes, beeps, tweets, the list grows everyday. Set the phone down, get up from the screens, and take a little time to get out in nature. Don't think you have nature because you live in a concrete jungle, go hit a park, go walk and

peer heaveneward and take in the majesty of the real world, the outdoors, small or great.

Or take a daycation or a drive to a nearby state or national park and take in some of this world's majesty. Go it solo and enjoy the solitude and bask in your adventure, or assemble your squad and create new joyous memories, or if you have a dog they can make great trail buddies too.

Pets have a way of reminding us how to let go and be totally present in the moment. When you return to civilization, your mind and body will feel clear and focused.

8. Release stored tension. When you feel your shoulders tightening from sitting in traffic or staring at a computer, you can ease your own stress in five minutes or less. With your right hand, tuck your thumb under your fingers and curl your fingers down toward your palm, making a soft fist.

Rest your right elbow in your left hand and use your right fist to gently tap on your left shoulder and upper arm. Tap gently, focusing more on the upward movement of your hand than the downward strike, and avoid any prominent bones.

Repeat on your other side. Once finished, take a few deep, cleansing breaths and feel your shoulders relaxed and tingling.

11 • WAYS TO ELIMINATE STRESS

It can seem sometimes as if there's nothing you can do about your stress level. Your brain doing what it does, says things like... "The bills are piling up and aren't going to stop coming,' or 'there will never be more hours in the day for all of the errands I need to run, and my career and family responsibilities must be done or calamity will strike'. It's hard to drown out that everpresent voice in our heads, processing, thinking, reminding us of the important and the trivial.

Most of us get so accustomed to stress in our daily lives, that it becomes like a second nature and we do not know what it is that caused the stress in the first place. Often, what causes stress are the very thoughts that we are thinking.

When we experience stress it is because our thoughts are aligned with a potential consequence, the negative, instead of the outcome which we desire.

We are operate out of fear. It is easy to explain this difference using an example of two athletes. One athlete enjoys their sport and is confident in themselves and their ability. So, when this athlete steps up to the starting line, their thoughts are focused on winning and the fun of the race. They are focused on the positive, the emotions flooding this athlete's system are ones of anticipation and excitement and enjoyment of their sport. The second athlete may be struggling with their confidence in their ability or belief in self and so when they step up to the starting line, their thoughts are not focused on "winning", but instead they focus on not "not losing". They focus on the negative outcome, on the possibility of losing and the consequences of such an outcome. This will cause the emotions flooding this athlete's system to be those of stress and anxiety and can lead to a lack of enjoyment in their sport like they normally would without the presence of stress.

The stress response floods your body with chemicals that prepare you for "fight or flight." In other words, it prepares you for consequences, we've evolved to have this response to ensure survival. The problem is we live in a world, a reality, we have a part in creating, based on the thoughts in our heads. We've probably all heard terms or phrases like 'The power of positive thinking' or describing someone as 'glass half-full'.

The emotions we feel including stress affect the types of experiences we are creating for ourselves in our lives. If you are mentally focused on undesired results or negativity you will feel stress and if the stress becomes chronic, you can inevitably end up creating the very undesired results you are trying to avoid.

It has been said that this is an attraction based universe. Meaning whatever you say "no" to, you are attracting into your experience and whatever you say "yes" to, you are attracting into your experience.

Attraction based in that what we give attention to we give power to. You can't say "no" to a thing without focusing on it. And an attraction-based universe says that whatever you focus on will come to be in the physical universe-That our thoughts manifest our reality.

Can we say for sure that this is how it all works – no, but the truth of the matter is that you have a lot more control than you might think. In fact, the simple realization that you're in control of your life and that you control your life with your thoughts is a foundation of stress management.

Managing stress is all about taking charge. And making how you feel and your emotions a priority of your life. Reducing stress is about taking charge of your thoughts, your environment, and the way you deal with problems. You don't need to fear stress, we need to learn to use it to our advantage.

Recognize it within yourself, see it as a beneficial red flag to signal that you may need to adjust your way of thinking or habits.

Here are a few more tools and ideas to help you curb the stresses in your life.

1. Identify your sources of stress as well as the unhealthy coping strategies you may be use to avoid stress.
Examine your habits, routines, attitudes, and excuses.

Do you define stress as an integral part of your work or home life by identifying with beliefs like "Things are always crazy around here" or as a part of your personality by aligning with beliefs like "I am just a naturally anxious person", or "I am just a worrier... that's all".

Do you have the habit of explaining away stress as temporary when it is not? Do you say things like "I just have a million things going on right now" despite the fact that you can't remember the last time you took a breather?

Do you blame your stress on other people or outside events instead of recognizing the damaging beliefs or thought patterns which attract people and events which increase your stress levels into your life? Do you view your stress as entirely normal and therefore unexceptional?

Until you accept responsibility for the role you play in creating or maintaining stress, your stress level will remain outside your control. Do you practice coping strategies which temporarily reduce stress but cause more damage in the long run such as:

- Smoking
- Drinking
- Overeating or under eating
- Trying to avoid stressors by spending hours in front of the TV or computer
- Withdrawing from friends, family, and activities
- Using pills or drugs to relax

- Escaping by sleeping too much
- Procrastinating
- Filling up every minute of the day with things to do so as to avoid facing problems.

Or...

- Taking out your stress on others (lashing out, angry outbursts, physical violence)

It is very important when you are plotting your course to where you want to be in life, to first be honest with yourself about where you are currently. Realize that where you are is just where you are. There is nothing keeping you there but you. And recognize that you not only want your life to feel better but you also are committed to finding a way to feel better.

2. Change the way you are thinking.

How you think has a profound effect on your emotional and physical well-being. Each time you think a negative thought about yourself or your life, your body reacts as if it were in the throes of a tension-filled situation.

If you think positive thoughts about yourself and your life, your body will react by releasing chemicals which make you feel good. Work to eliminate words such as "always," "never," "should," and "must." from your vocabulary. These definitive statements are very conducive to thoughts which are self-defeating and create stress.

Don't try to control the uncontrollable. Many things in life are beyond our control (things like the behavior of other people for example). Rather than stressing out about the things you can't control, focus on the things that you can control. The only things we have real control over in our lives are our own thoughts.

The more control we learn to have over our own thoughts, the more power we will have in our lives. Our thoughts are the one thing no one else can choose for us. The more power we feel that we have in life, the less stress we will feel.

You cannot feel free and relaxed when you continue to focus on things which make you feel powerless and which you cannot control. So, learn to let go of them.

Reframe problems. Learn to think positively by practicing thinking thoughts about yourself and your life that feel better to you when you think them. Try to view stressful situations from a more positive perspective.

For example, rather than panicking about a traffic jam, look at it as an opportunity to pause and regroup, listen to your favorite radio station, or enjoy some alone time. When stress is getting you down, take a moment to reflect on all the things you appreciate in your life, including your own positive qualities and gifts. This simple strategy can help you keep things in perspective.

Look at the big picture. Learn to view your stressful situation from a different perspective. Ask yourself how important it will be in the long run. Will it matter in a month? Will it matter in a year? Is it really worth getting upset over? If the answer is no, focus your time and energy elsewhere.

Perfectionism is a major source of avoidable stress. Stop setting yourself up for failure by demanding perfection. Perfection is a completely subjective concept. Perfection is in the eye of the beholder. Set reasonable standards for yourself and others. And learn to love yourself the way you are instead of basing your worthiness on what you present or produce in life.

Many of us are goal oriented. We see happiness as an end result. A destination we get to and then the journey stops. The truth is it never stops. You will never "get it all done". The process of living is one of continual evolution, when we achieve something we desire, we do not stop desiring.

Instead, we desire something else. This is the way life was intended to be. So, the point of life is enjoying the process (every aspect of the process). Sometimes if you just accept that you will never get it all done and there will always be more you are reaching for, you can let yourself off the hook of trying to get everything finished right here and now as soon as you possibly can.

3. Figure out what makes you happy.

By the time many of us are dealing with stress, we are standing in adulthood surrounded by a life which has not been deliberately created. Instead, it has been created by default.

This means that we have based our goals and desires not off of what makes us happy. But instead off of what satisfies the priorities of others (especially authority figures in our early life and society as a whole).

Many of us have lost touch with what makes us happy. The risk of placing value on what makes you happy and who you really are often feels like the risk of not being loved for what is real about yourself. It can also feel like the risk of being seen as a failure by others (which is a threat to most people's sense of self worth) so it is easy to see how placing value on what makes you truly happy can be a very frightening proposition.

But until you reveal your true desires and what truly makes you happy, it is not possible to be truly happy. If you have lost touch with what makes you happy, one of the best ways to get back in touch with it, is to think back to your natural inclinations as a child.

Make a long list of things you knew you loved when you were a child. Make a list of your natural talents as a child and try to remember what you wanted to be when you grew up.

Now, after you make that list, make sure to ask yourself why. Why did you love those things? Why did you possess those natural talents? Why did you want to grow up to be those things?

Then ask yourself "do I still enjoy and practice these things?" If not...why? Can I remember what caused me to stop? Was it because of someone else? Do I remember how it felt to stop doing those things? And then, take step forward by trying some of these things you once loved to do... again.

From here, fast forward. Ask yourself what your favorite part of your entire life was so far and why that particular point was your favorite part of your life. Get as detailed as you can in order to discover the true reason you enjoyed it so much.

And after that, ask yourself what you enjoy about the life you are living in now? What am I passionate about in my life currently? Have I devoted those things to the back burner, or are they the primary focus of my life?

This process will help you to understand what it is that you truly enjoy separate of your conditioned and logical brain which (being mechanical in nature) has often been taught to minimize feeling states such as joy and passion.

Finding your own personal idea of happiness, and this is very individual, is an incredibly important component of stress reduction, as we strive for and reach this happiness we reduce and push those stresses out of our experience.

4. Equip yourself with tools that work for YOU to reduce stress.

There are many sources and products which exist worldwide whose sole purpose is to help you to reduce stress. So, seek them out. Begin by making a list of things which you can already identify that help you to reduce stress. When stress comes up, get in the habit of going to the list and picking something off of the list to do.

Set out to learn and practice relaxation techniques. The relaxation response brings your system back into balance. It deepens your breathing, reducing stress hormones, slows down your heart rate and blood pressure, and relaxes your muscles.

In addition to its calming physical effects, research shows that the relaxation response also increases energy and focus, combats illness, relieves aches and pains, heightens problem-solving abilities, and boosts motivation and productivity.

Relaxation techniques may include things such as Emotional Freedom Technique, deep breathing, visualization, progressive muscle relaxation, meditation, yoga, tai chi, massage, stretching or aromatherapy.

5. Make your physical health a priority.

The body is an incredibly reflective instrument. When the mind is thinking negative, stressful thoughts, those thoughts are reflected in the body. But it is also true that when the body is kept in a state of negativity and stress, that stress and negativity is reflected in the mind. So, it is very helpful to take control of your physical health.

Exercise Regularly. Exercise does not have to be a source of more stress. In fact it can be a great stress reducer if you can find an exercise that you enjoy doing instead of simply exercising for the sake of exercise.

Physical activity helps to increase the production of your brain's feel-good neurotransmitters, called endorphins. Endorphins are natural pain killers and they make you feel "happy".

They are responsible for the well-known "runner's high". Exercise forces tense muscles (through use), to release their state of tension. Exercise can also be like a meditation in motion. You'll often find that you've forgotten the day's irritations and concentrated purely on your body's movements when you are exercising. And it helps you release pent up stressful energy.

As you begin to regularly shed your daily tensions through movement and physical activity, you may find that this focus on a single task, and the resulting energy and optimism, can help you remain calm and clear in everything that you do. Exercise also can improve your quality of sleep.

Eat healthy, well-balanced meals. You are what you eat. A nutritious diet can counteract the impact of stress, by reinforcing the immune system and lowering blood pressure.

Comfort foods (like mashed potatoes) have been shown to boost levels of serotonin, a calming brain chemical. Other foods can reduce levels of cortisol and adrenaline (stress hormones that take a toll on the body).

Stressed people tend to gain weight and make food choices which are not conducive to health. There is a lot of information available from experts on diets which specifically reduce stress as well as many herbal supplements that have been shown to diminish stress.

Go looking for them and try to implement the suggestions. You will be surprised by the results. It is important that you don't rely on sugar, caffeine, alcohol or other drugs to reduce stress. Relying on such things not only creates physical or mental dependency, it harms your body in the long run.

Get enough rest and sleep. Sleep deprivation is chronic in our culture. Sleep deprivation is one of the chief aggravators of stress. Lack of sleep increases levels of cortisol, a stress hormone.

Sleep deprivation also affects the immune system (depleting certain cells needed to destroy viruses and cancerous cells), it promotes the growth of fat instead of muscle, and speeds up the aging process.

Your body needs time to recover from stressful events. Adequate sleep fuels your mind, as well as your body. Feeling tired will increase your stress because it may cause you to think irrationally. When you are tired, you are less patient and easily agitated which can increase stress.

And then, to make matters worse, you will not have the energy to deal with the stress. Most adults need 7-8 hours of sleep per night. Start to make sleep a priority. Start to see it as a necessity not a luxury.

6. Learn to manage your time more effectively.

In this physical dimension, we lead linear lives. No matter how skilled any of us may think we are at multi-tasking, when it comes to action, we can only be in one place at one time. What's more, we can only really do one task well in each moment.

For the average man or woman, day to day life is a whirlwind of frantic activity. Life is composed of rushing from one task to another while still not really accomplishing anything of value at the end of the day. It is therefore very useful to learn to manage our time more effectively.

Using time more effectively helps to eliminate stress by making order of chaos. It is very helpful to reduce stress by getting organized. No one can think clearly when they are surrounded in a physical environment which is chaotic. So begin by cleaning and organizing your environment.

A mental environment which is cluttered is conducive to stress and ineffective time management as well. One way to combat this kind of chaos is to learn how to write lists and then prioritize. Set clear goals and break your goals down into discreet steps. To be effective, you need to decide what tasks are urgent and important and to focus on those.

Devote the majority of your time to the most important tasks. Trying to remember everything in your head is a recipe for stress. When you do not have to worry about remembering everything (because it is written down) you will be more able to accomplish the things and also your stress levels will diminish.

Writing lists helps you identify important objectives, helps you order your thoughts, helps you prioritize, helps you see the big picture, saves time, helps you feel in control, helps you track your progression, and makes you much less likely to forget to do things.

Identify areas of your life where you are wasting time and come up with a plan to reduce them. It may help to even enlist the help of others to help you stick to it. It may help some people to also develop a routine so they can know what to focus on when. One useful way to develop a routine and thereby eliminate wasted time is to use a time log.

To do this, make up a chart for the next seven days divided into half hour intervals starting the log at the time you get up and finish it at the time you go to bed. Write down what you do during each half hour of the day for the next seven days.

Choose a typical week. At the end of the week examine your time log and ask yourself the following questions: Are there any periods that I could use more productively?

At what time of day do I do my most effective work? (Some people are most alert in the morning, whilst others concentrate best during the afternoon or evening). Schedule your most important tasks for these times of day. Eliminate wasted time by replacing it with activities that are conducive to a more fulfilling, enjoyable and productive lifestyle.

7. Express your emotions.

We currently live in a society that does not understand the value and role of emotions. We live in a society which also tends to promote repression instead of expression. But unexpressed emotions affect your life. Start to label your emotions. This will help you to identify them when they come up. Emotions are transient.

They will dissipate as they are expressed. The only type of emotion that lingers is repressed emotion. If something or someone is bothering you, voice your concerns in an open and respectful way.

If you don't voice your feelings, not only will resentment will build but the situation will likely remain the same. You may want to use physical expression as a route to releasing emotions.

Make sure you choose a physical activity that will not harm another person or yourself. Some good ways to express anger and stress include punching pillows, screaming into pillows, taking out a pen and paper and writing what you feel, painting or drawing what you feel, hitting the ground with a stick, popping balloons, taking a kickboxing class, going for a run or trying to get yourself to cry.

It will feel good to get the tears flowing. It will surprise you how much better this will make you feel. The emotions will no longer be like a wall preventing you from moving forward if you express them in a healthy way.

8. Keep your life simple and learn how to say no.

Keeping life simple isn't always easy. Simplicity is especially hard to attain in this fast paced century which we are currently living in. We often lose track of why we are doing what we are doing. We go so fast and create such busy, complicated lives that we forget that we have control of our lives. Instead it feels like our lives are running us.

The human ego loves complexity because it measures worth in quantity instead of quality. It also bases it's self off of comparison with others. Our ego relies on fear to protect itself and complexity is a great place to hide. Simplicity therefore, requires dedication.

Begin the quest towards simplicity by asking yourself honestly what areas of your life you feel need to be simplified. Identify what is holding you back from simplifying them. Eliminate the clutter and unnecessary aspects of your life.

Get rid of stuff you don't use. Stop trying to please everyone. Instead, simply do what you intuitively feel that you know is right. Finish one project before you start another.

Dedicate more time with what is really important in your life. Don't buy stuff you don't need. While it is perfectly fine to desire a life of wealth, as well as work on creating it in your life, there is almost nothing worse for adding to stress levels than living beyond your means. This will set up a dynamic of focusing on the amount of money you don't have. Aim at living below your means.

This does not mean you should live in an attitude of denying yourself what you desire. It simply means making decisions that ensure that you will end up with excess and therefore be focusing on the feeling of abundance instead of lack. Consolidate everything you can find to consolidate.

Permit yourself to enjoy the present moments of your life (the now). It is important also to know your limits and to stick to them. In both your personal or professional life, refuse to accept added responsibilities, especially when you're close to reaching goals. Taking on more than you can handle instantly gives rise to stress.

Many of us fear saying no. We think that to say no is selfish. And we often feel as if saying yes is the only way to earn the love of others. But, love which must be earned is not real love. And it is not selfish to ensure our own happiness because when we are happy and feeling stress free, we have the energy and resources to devote to others.

When we are unhappy and feeling stressed, we often become ill and have no energy to devote to others anyway. When you say no to a new commitment which would add stress to your life, you're honoring your existing obligations and ensuring that you'll be able to devote quality time to them.

Burying yourself in commitments ensures that you will begin to feel just that buried. Saying no may not be the easiest thing to do. But sometimes it is the necessary ingredient for practicing self care as well as eliminating stress from your life.

9. Make time for fun and relaxation by finding healthy ways to relax and recharge and giving yourself permission to do so.

The sad fact about stress is that most people who experience stress have their priorities backwards. For example, they may think that perfection is the most important thing in life or that responsibility is the most important thing in life.

What they fail to recognize is the very reason for which they seek out perfection or responsibility. And the reason is this... they think they will feel better when they produce something which is perfect or when they are responsible than they would in the absence of perfection or responsibility.

It is therefore important for those suffering from stress to realize that the sole reason for doing those things they "have to do" comes from the motivation of feeling better, in other words happiness. This means that all people most especially those who suffer from stress would do very well to cut to the chase and make the priority of their lives (their true motivation) how they feel.

It is important for the highest priority in a person's life to be none other than... happiness. The things which each specific person finds enjoyable and relaxing varies but some ideas for healthy ways to relax and recharge include:

- Call a good friend
- Spend time outside
- Take a bath
- Sweat out tension with a good workout
- Write in a journal
- Savor a warm cup of tea

- Make yourself one of your comfort foods
- Spend time with a pet (pets have been shown to dramatically reduce stress)
- Get a massage.
- Play a game
- Read a book
- Drive to a place with an amazing view
- Listen to music
- Watch a comedy movie
- Connect with others. Spending time with positive people who enhance your life. A strong support system will buffer you from the negative effects of stress

One of the greatest ways to reduce stress in your life is to make sure that you do something you enjoy and which recharges your engine every day. It does not have to be done alone. In fact, these kinds of activities can be used to re charge the entire family.

10. Never underestimate the power of laughing.

Seek out and create opportunities which will make you laugh.

It turns out that laughter may just be the best medicine of all. You have probably noticed that laughter is infectious. Laughter binds people together and increases happiness and intimacy. Humor lightens your burdens and inspires your hopes.

Humor helps you to shift perspective and paints things in a less threatening light. It enhances resiliency and it also triggers healthy physical responses in the body. Laughter has been shown to strengthen the immune system. Laughter decreases stress hormones and increases immune cells and infection-fighting antibodies, thereby improving your resistance to disease.

Like exercise, laughter triggers the release of endorphins, the body's natural feel-good chemicals. Endorphins promote an overall sense of well-being and can even relieve pain. Laughter has been shown to improve the function of blood vessels and increase blood flow which leads to improved heart health.

In studies, it has also been shown that a good, hearty laugh leaves your muscles relaxed for up to 45 minutes. Laughter protects you from the plethora of damaging effects which stress can cause to the body and the mind. It is fun and it also does not cost anything.

So, when you are trying to eliminate stress from your life, try to indulge your laughter as much as you possibly can.

Allow and seek out avenues for it to surface. You can even begin with a smile. Smiling is the beginning of laughter. It too is contagious. It too released endorphins. Seek out ways to develop your own sense of humor.

Seek out that which is funny to you, whether it is renting a funny movie, calling up the friend who always makes you laugh or developing an arsenal of jokes to tell. As laughter becomes an integrated part of your life you will be taken to a mental space where you can view the world from a more relaxed, positive, and balanced perspective.

Many of us have the self defeating belief that everything that is worth having is hard won. But this belief ensures that we are going about life in the wrong way. We should approach things with much more ease. Doing things the hard way causes stress, and stress, in actuality, keeps the desired results from you.

If you are brave enough to make feeling good the primary priority of your life and then take the steps necessary to enable your own joy as well as reduce stress levels, you can find yourselves living the life that you want to live. A Life that feels good to be living, that brings you joy, health, happiness, and fulfilment.

12 • DEEP BREATHING FOR ANXIETY AND STRESS MANAGEMENT

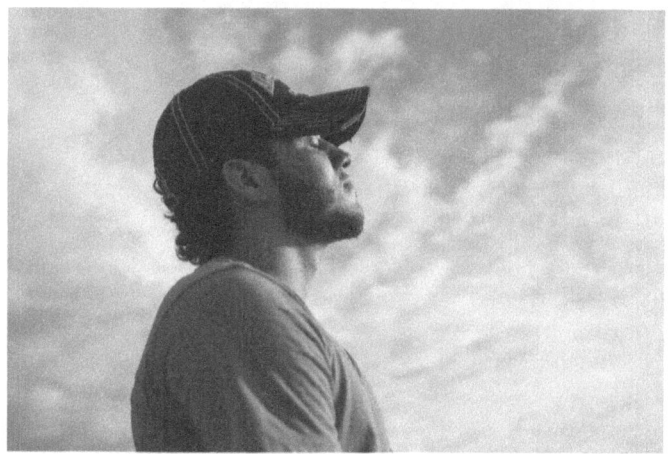

Deep breathing is one of the single most important habits you can develop to improve and maintain health. You've been breathing all your life but seldom do we take the time to cultivate good breathing habits. The box breathing we covered can really work wonders for stress management and reducing anxiety attacks. But what about breathing in general, how can we improve our breathing to improve our overall outcomes?

Your main focus with deep breathing is getting fresh air into your lungs. As your heart pumps blood, the first place it goes is into your lungs to become oxygenated. After your lungs, your blood transports oxygen throughout your body.

This helps to maintain healthy pH (acidity/alkalinity) and provides critical oxygen to all your organs and bodily tissues. Deep breathing has a multitude of beneficial effects. One of the most immediate benefits is stress management.

Long, slow, even, deep breaths can stop an anxiety attack. Two or three minutes of deep breathing can provide stress relief for rush hour traffic, a hectic day of work, or holiday shopping.

Additional benefits are clearer thinking (oxygen to the brain), balanced blood pressure, and increased detoxification. Your lungs play a very important role in overall health and everything about deep breathing is lung friendly.

One great habit is to take 10 long, slow, deep breaths before going into grocery or department stores. After you are done shopping and get back into your car, gently close your eyes and visualize walking in a forest, gazing at the ocean, or anything else you find relaxing.

While visualizing, take a few deep breaths. If other thoughts come, acknowledge them and bring your attention back to your breathing. You'll feel an amazing sense of peace and harmony within minutes. This is an excellent stress management technique.

Another simple breathing technique is to take a few deep breaths at trigger points throughout your day: When you first wake up in the morning, take 10 long, slow, deep breaths. Repeat at bedtime, after meals, and before going to bed.

Additionally, any time during your day you feel stress or anxiety, take a few seconds to breathe deeply. Practicing these breathing techniques at each of these trigger points will cultivate healthy breathing habits throughout your day.

When deep breathing, inhale through your nose and exhale through your mouth. This provides more effective utilization of the oxygen. The key is breathe long, slow, and deep. Inhale fully and exhale completely. You'll find over time a significant reduction in anxiety attacks and an improvement in stress management.

13 • MINDFULNESS TO MANAGE ANXIETY AND STRESS

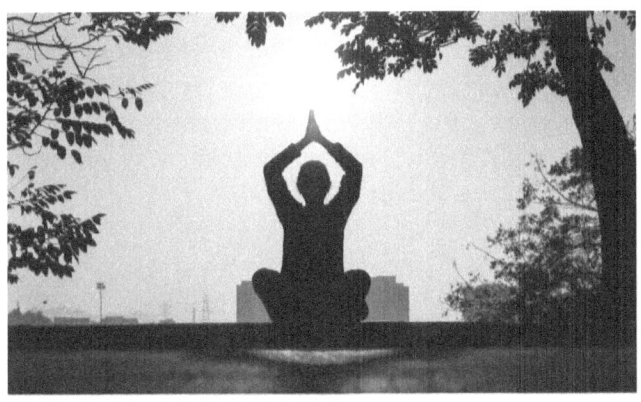

Mindfulness meditation increases your level of self-awareness. It helps you get in touch with what is happening around you and slows down your reaction to it. In fact it takes you deeper into a relaxed state where you are calm and there is no fear, anxiety or stress. It can improve your mental function and reduce impulsiveness.

Below is an effective method. It is recommended that you read this slowly 2-3 times just before doing it. Even while you are reading it you will start noticing your breathing pattern.

Breathing in and out

1.	Sit in a comfortable chair or on a cushion on the floor. Choose a chair that will straighten your back. If you choose to sit on the floor, make sure that you are sitting on a cushion that will support and lift your back side.

It is important to remain motionless during meditation. Even if you feel the urge to move in order to adjust any part of your body, do not act on it.

At first you might find this difficult, but as this process continues, you will be able to control that impulse. These are automatic impulses that your mind creates. You will be aware of it, but you will not act on it. In a way you are gaining greater control over your mind.

2. As you sit still notice your breathing. You can close your eyes or not, whatever you are comfortable with because it does not matter. As you focus on your breathing you will notice how slower and deeper your breathing has become.

Silently say to yourself "inhale" as you breathe in and "exhale" as you breathe out. When you notice your mind wandering - and it will - gently bring it back to your breathing.

3. Now you can stop saying "inhale" and "exhale", just keep on breathing slowly and deeply. You might notice the sensations of the breath flowing in and out of your nose or mouth. You might sense the belly or chest expanding as you breathe in, and deflating as you breathe out.

As you breathe in and breathe out your body will go deeper and deeper into a relaxed state. Push back your inner dialogues to the back of your mind and keep your focus on the breathing.

Keep doing this for as long as you can. Start with 5-6 breaths and keep on increasing with time. Most people give up because they try to do it for 10-15 mins and their mind wanders a lot. They get frustrated and give up. Start with 2 minutes. And remember your mind will wander, your job is to bring it back gently to your breathing.

As you keep doing this on a daily basis, you will become calmer and thoughtful. Your stress levels will come down and you will be able see through and manage your anxiety period.

14 • LIVING WELL AT ANY AGE

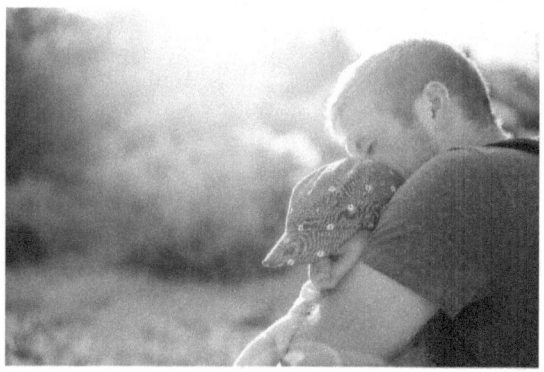

Our 20's

At this age, stress is a well-used word. Poorly managed stress is a threat to both physical and mental health, work safety and productivity. Stress continues to challenge every day.

The battle against fatigue is also ongoing. The importance of a balanced diet and exercise in maintaining energy levels at times when the demands on performance are continually high is well documented.

Fiber, good fats, low GI carbohydrates and wise protein choices are fundamental in energy production. Additionally, magnesium is a wonderful tension reliever, and works well to restore restful sleep.

Our 30's

Working hard and planning a family places a different emphasis on the nutritional requirements for each partner. A variety of demands on your time and resources can lift stress levels to a new high. Stress in all its guises, causes an increased demand for a range of essential and complementary nutritional factors.

Our 40's

'Middle age' is a time when some of the common chronic diseases such as elevated blood pressure and diabetes are noticed (if not earlier). Demands on time and additional financial pressures can lead to poor dietary choices and less exercise.

High stress levels lead to increases in inflammatory markers, resulting in oxidative damage to blood vessels. Regular health assessments by a medical provider are important-DON'T just rely on webMD and google!

Men can be poor observers of health issues, but are lucky to have the moderating and wise opinions of their partners, as their health can often be pushed into the background.

Children are keen mimics of our behavior patterns, so regular mealtimes with the family form a wonderful base on which they will build their own impressions of food types, appropriate mealtime behavior and their ability to communicate well.

Time for adequate exercise and relaxation is hard to find, but must be part of your healthy routine. Stretching before exercise and suitable warm down procedures will ensure minimal injury interruptions.

Magnesium is a great mineral to relax tired and aching muscles, and encourage restful sleep. Maintain and protect "me time" if you can. Rest is a wonderful tonic for stress, and demands on your time.

Our 50's Those good habits we have put into place are paying huge health dividends now. As an acknowledgment that our hormones are changing, there are some other health challenges to address. Alterations in hormone levels are reflected by interrupted sleep, mood fluctuations and an awareness that the adolescents in the family are becoming independent (or at least we hope they are.).

Food choices and healthy recipes continue to be important. More omega-3 in the form of oily fish plays an important part in hormone support, skin moisture content and elasticity, and concentration. It also plays a role in cardiovascular health and as an antiinflammatory in joint pain.

Sleep can be the biggest challenge. Make sure your sleep pattern is structured and consistent. Start to relax well before you expect sleep to overtake you. Find the best ways to induce drowsiness in your own particular instance - everybody is different. However, the need for sleep as a recovery aid is fundamental to emotional, physical and mental health.

Take a 50+ multivitamin each day, along with additional calcium in the most soluble forms. Good digestion can be encouraged by addressing gut issues like bloating or constipation.

Our 60's

The ability to move well, use your brain to its maximum potential and have minimal risk of chronic disease are the ultimate goals. Regular assessments by a trusted health professional ensure that small alterations will keep you well.

There is much truth in the adage "Use it or lose it". This applies especially to your brain and your joints. The brain relies on good levels of nutrients to function correctly, along with adequate hydration.

Calcium is an important component of bone health, preferably using a calcium type which is easily digested by levels of gastric acid which lessen as we age, and which are often compromised by medicines.

Calcium rich foods and vitamin D are important considerations too, because it's been shown that food sources as well as supplementation are the best solution to bone health.

Moving our joints without discomfort seems simple enough, but as we age, many years of wear and tear are reflected by stiffness and inflammation. Glucosamine is an excellent way of supporting joint structure and relieving any tendency to inflammation, and is also safe for long term use.

Vegetarian options are available if you have a seafood sensitivity. Additionally, omega-3 fatty acids available as fish oil or krill oil, allow a constant supply of anti-inflammatory action to safely circulate throughout your system, settling inflamed blood vessels, digestive linings and worn joints.

Eat well, enjoy life, maximize vitality and use appropriate nutritional supplements to enhance your lifestyle.

15 • HOW CAN WE DIFFUSE A STRESSFUL MOMENT OR PANIC ATTACK?

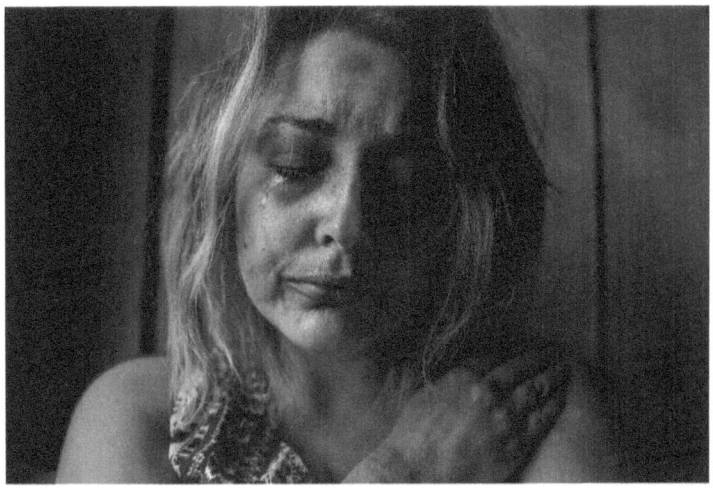

First off it's important to note what a panic attack actually is, that way you know what it is that you are going to stop. A panic attack is at its most basic level, your body reacting to an outside source in a way that it does not know how to properly react to, much like an allergy.

All an allergy is, is your body deciding that something harmless, like flower pollen, or dog hair, is actually harmful to you and it activates its own built in systems to get rid of the object. In that respect, a panic attack is your body activating the fight or flight mechanisms in a situation when it does not need too.

Fortunately, a panic attack is not dangerous, like a bee sting allergy, or a peanut allergy. That being said panic attacks are very uncomfortable and not a pleasant experience.

One personal note that I would like to state before we go on with what to do when having a panic attack, is that panic attacks are very common and very normal. Almost everyone has them at one point or another in their life, there is nothing wrong with you and you are not alone.

When I first had a panic attack I felt like it was something that only I was having and that it was something wrong with me. But I realized, it was not my fault, and could take steps to help myself through the attack if it happened again. That being said let's get started on helping you get through your panic attacks.

Sudden Onset Panic Attack:

Sudden onset panic attack is a classification for a panic attack that comes seemingly out of nowhere without any warning.

First off, remind yourself that this is your body reacting to nothing, it's like an allergy. The reason you have to make sure this is on your mind, is so that you don't try to find the reason you're having this panic attack. If you start to search for a reason or an external object that may be causing this you will only prolong your attack.

Second, try to observe what you are feeling. I know this sounds unusual so let me explain. When you have a panic attack keep track of what you are feeling physically, literally list in your head or out loud, "my pulse is racing, I feel like I am being watched, My chest is tightening."

It is very important to note that you should not react to the attack, you have to take on the mindset of a person who is observing, like a reporter, you are to report, not interfere.

The reason behind this is simple, trying to stop a panic attack will only prolong it, concentrating on making it stop will only cause you more stress about it not stopping fast enough. If you let it happen, and I know that doesn't sound pleasant, but if you let it happen and monitor what you are feeling it will end itself.

By observing it, you give your mind something to do, so you stop trying to end your panic attack, and you let it end on its own. You distract yourself from the stessor by observing and paying attention to what's happening to you at that time.

Another additional part that might help is to monitor the changes in what you feel, and say to yourself, "the feeling is the same" or "the feeling is changing" every ten seconds or so. Doing this has helped me to take the major edge off of my panic attacks and shorten them from as long as hour, to as short as only a minute.

The third step, once you start to feel the major part of the panic attack subside is to remember to breathe. Now, I don't mean hyperventilate, I mean breathe. Take a deep breathe in and count how long it takes you to inhale. Most people can do it between 5 and 8 seconds, however if you can do more great.

Then exhale slowly, try to see if you can let your exhale last twice as long as you're inhale. So if you can inhale for 5 seconds see if you can make your exhale 10 seconds. If you can't that is perfectly ok, don't stress yourself out about this just look at it as an experiment to see if you can do it. If you start to feel light headed or dizzy, take a few regular breaths.

Once you start to feel yourself calming down, and your breathing seems natural and you feel the panic attack is subsiding, grab a piece of paper and a pen, not a computer, and write down your thoughts on paper. It doesn't matter what you write down, just start to write by hand.

The reason for this is that typing uses less muscles and parts of your brain then writing, so if you sit down and write by hand, you will occupy more of your body and mind and allow it to relax.

It doesn't matter what you write, you can write about your day, what you want to do tomorrow, what you had for dinner, you can even write a paper about how crazy this idea sounds, it doesn't matter.

If, and only if you have something specific that you think is on your mind that caused the panic attack you can write about that specific thing but only if you can do so calmly.

Finally, and this may be the hardest part of this, find someone to talk to. You don't have to talk about the panic attack or what caused it unless you feel comfortable doing so, but find another human being to talk to, it can be in person, on the phone, over Skype it doesn't matter.

It is however better if it's in a method where you can hear the person so try to avoid Instant messaging and texting.

So, in summary, for a sudden onset panic attack the steps are as follows:

Step 1: Remind yourself that this is your body reacting to nothing, and that YOU ARE SAFE.

Step 2: Try to observe what you are feeling, don't try to stop it, let it burn itself out naturally.

Step 3: Take slow deep breaths to relax yourself, breathe normally if you feel dizzy or lightheaded.

Step 4: Sit down and write with a pen and paper your thoughts on whatever topic comes to mind.

Step 5: Talk to another human being for a while, just so you can get other parts of your mind working.

Stopping a panic attack before it starts:

Although it's important to know how to stop a panic attack once it occurs its always better to stop it before it starts wouldn't you agree?

The key to stopping a panic attack that is just starting to come on is to distract your mind and your body so it doesn't activate the fight or flight reflex. Unlike dealing with a sudden onset panic attack there are no steps to how to stop this but here are a few suggestions.

Go for a walk. Walking is great exercise, and it will give your body something useful to do with the adrenaline that it's pumping into your system. You don't have to walk fast, a slow peaceful walk will do just fine.

If you don't like walking do any kind of physical activity that you enjoy, ride your bike, play basketball, go shopping, play your favorite Wii sports game, or even clean.

It doesn't matter, just make sure you mentally focus on the activity, not the panic attack. If you focus on the panic attack it will stick around, if you focus on the activity it will burn itself out and you'll get your exercise in for the day.

Journal your thoughts. Like before, grab a piece of paper and a pen and start writing down what you're thinking about. It doesn't have to be related to the panic attack, in fact if writing it down starts to make you feel it more start to write about something else.

There is no wrong thing to write about in this situation. Just write, the activity of writing will occupy your mind and body enough for the panic attack to subside before it starts.

Distract yourself. I know it sounds kind of sarcastic, but it will actually work. Just give yourself something else to focus on and let your body burn out the feelings of the panic attack. Generally it's best if you give yourself something to do that is physical, or interactive. Like talking to a friend, cleaning, or playing a video game. Reading a book may work for you as well.

The key is to remember to not focus on the panic attack, and if what you're doing doesn't work don't get upset or stressed, just say to yourself "This was a good idea but I think I will do something else now" and that's it. Half of beating a panic attack is keeping control of your own thoughts so they don't run away from you.

The last thing I am going to suggest is meditation. This actually would work better if you practice this for five minutes a day when you are not having a panic attack.

That way when you think you may have one this will be a calming practice your body is familiar with, and can help you to switch your body from fight or flight mode into something more relaxed and centered.

The easiest way to meditate for a beginner is just to sit down in a comfortable spot, for most people that's a comfortable chair, you can sit on the floor cross legged if you can do so comfortably but most people, myself included, cannot and it's not required.

Once you are in a comfortable position, take a deep breath, and close your eyes. Then simply observe your breathing. By observe I mean watch, listen, and be aware of how your body feels. Don't try to slow your breathing down, don't try to control your breathing. Just pay attention to it.

Notice how your body moves when you breathe, does your chest rise and fall, or does your stomach rise and fall? What does your breathing sound like? Do you breathe through your nose or mouth? Can you feel the air moving through your throat or not?

All you do is pay attention to the actions of your breathing, and nothing else. If your mind starts to wander you can let it wander, that's ok, I have found letting my mind wander during meditation is a great way to clear up excess mental clutter.

Once your done letting it wander just focus on your breathing again and you will go right back to your meditation.

It's important to note that meditation is a skill, like riding a bike, or playing basketball. The more you practice the better you become, and you shouldn't expect to sit down and become one with the universe in your first attempt.

But no matter what happens, just try to meditate for 5 minutes a day and then when you feel a panic attack about to happen just focusing on your breathing may be all you need to stop it from happening.

Prevention:

More important than dealing with a panic attack when it is occurring is to take steps to prevent them completely. Although not all panic attacks stem from a person's lifestyle certain lifestyle choices can help to prevent panic attacks in general.

For starters, try to limit or cut out caffeine, tobacco, and alcohol from your lifestyle. Many people think that tobacco and alcohol will help relax you, but in reality both substances will mess with your internal body chemistry and make you more susceptible to a panic attack.

Caffeine, which is a stimulant, makes you more energized as well as more tense, and tension can lead to a panic attack. So your first steps should be to limit or eliminate all caffeine, tobacco, and alcohol from your lifestyle. I know it may be hard but if it stops your panic attacks it will be worth it don't you think?

The next suggestion is to write your thoughts down on paper once a day. A lot of panic attacks can be caused by things that are on our minds but that we don't know how to deal with or how to express.

Journaling for just a few minutes a day about whatever thoughts come to mind can help you to express your emotions and prevent them from manifesting into a panic attack.

The same works for any dreams you may have, just write down what occurred in the dream and it can help you clear your mind. Another helpful tip is that if you have a situation in your life that is bothering you, write it down, and ask yourself the following questions as you are writing it down:

What did I do right? What could I have done more of? What should I have done less of? What should I have added? What should I have eliminated? Then let it go, remember the past exists only so we can learn from it. Learn and then relax it's over, you deserve better then to carry a painful situation with you.

The last suggestion that I have for prevention is a simple one, get enough rest. In general your average adult needs 8 hours of sleep a night, but only gets 5. That lack of sleep causes tension, exhaustion and a whole host of chemical imbalances in your body. Sleeping is what your body uses to repair itself, mentally, physically and emotionally.

So do whatever you have to do to get 8 hours of sleep a night, it may not be easy the first week or so and you may wake up before you get 8 hours, but stick with it, your body will thank you. And don't forget to try to meditate for just 5 minutes a day. Those 5 minutes will make a big difference in your life trust me.

I hope you have found the advice I have given on what to do when having a panic attack, and how to prevent them useful.

16 • BENEFITS OF MEDITATION FOR NATURAL STRESS RELIEF

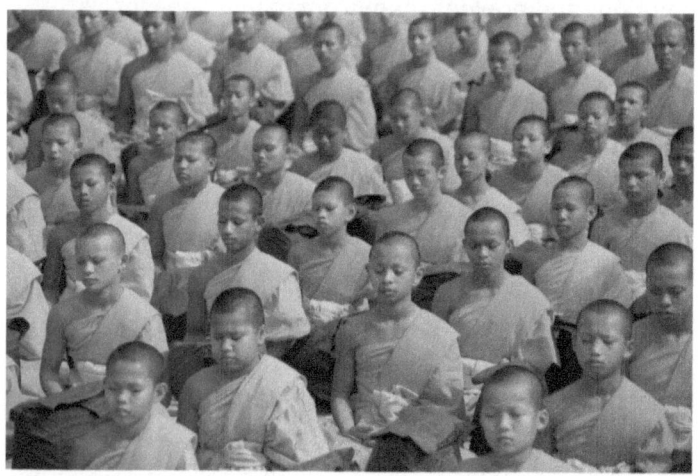

The practice of the ancient art of meditation has been known as an alternative and natural way to help heal the mind and body. In times of mental or physical stress, some people have used the powers of meditation to calm the mind and heal the body.

There is an intense connection between the mind and the body, and when one is in pain, the other usually suffers also.

Meditation can help begin a balance. Study has shown that meditation can have a helpful impact on the health of any human being, and these helpful effects are not partial to the body. When practiced consistently, it can greatly play a role to the health and well-being of not only the body but also the mind.

In today's hectic world, the use of meditation to relieve stress is widespread. In fact, as the practice of meditation gains in popularity, an increasing number of people from a CEO to a weary parent are including the exercise into their lifestyle.

In addition to using meditation to relieve stress, people practice it to guard against the many concerns upsetting the mind, and there is solid physiological proof to support its success in doing so.

With consistent use of meditation, you may experience some of the following helpful effects: A decrease in moodiness, irritability, depression and anxiety and an increase in happiness and emotional stability, feelings of rejuvenation and vitality, and greater creativity.

Many folks have also reported a large improvement in their ability to learn new things and preserve information. You may find that with consistent practice, meditation greatly improves your mental state and may add to a greater sense of spirituality. The spiritual person often sees the world in a uniquely positive way and is well-equipped to deal with life's challenges.

Though meditation is commonly known for its helpful relation to a person's mind and spirituality, the practice can also have beneficial physical effects.

Most likely, the first effect you will notice after continual practice of meditation is an increase in your flexibility which keeps your body responsive and functioning. There are other equally important changes to your physical self that you might notice such as the following:

Improvement in air flow to the lungs making it easier to breathe, a lowering in blood pressure, decreased levels of cortisol and lactate (two chemicals associated with stress), a lower heart rate, lowering of free radicals which can cause tissue damage, and a drop in cholesterol.

The consistent practice of meditation can also slow down the aging process - especially noticeable in the elderly who often convey major changes in their vitality.

The idea behind meditation is consciously relaxing the body and mind, through a variety of different techniques, each that have their own methods. Some methods want you to focus on certain things, like a quiet and relaxing spot on the beach, while others simply allow your mind to wander off, like sleeping, but in a different state of mind.

No matter which method you try, there are things that they all have in common. The first is that they involve deep breathing exercises. As we've discussed, breathing exercises get you to focus on something other than your stress. You are focusing on your breathing, counting the length of time you breathe in, and out.

The next thing all of these techniques have in common is that you need to do them every day, at least once a day, for twenty to thirty minutes. Some say you need more time, some say less. Many of us don't have that kind of time throughout the day, but if you can spend just ten or fifteen minutes twice a day, then a longer period before bed time, you will get the same benefits.

Common to all forms of meditation is that you need to be in a place with little or no distractions. You can use music if it helps you, and there are verbal things you can say to get you focused on meditation, rather than what is going on around you.

It is best to be sitting in a comfortable chair, with the lights dimmed. You don't want it dark, or the chair so comfortable that you fall asleep, because meditation is not sleep, but a higher state of consciousness.

Many businesses today are starting to realize the need for meditation in the work place, in order to keep stress levels down. Some companies even require employees to take a ten to twenty minute break just for meditation, and have rooms set aside for this purpose. The idea is that it's more productive to do this, than the time lost from employees getting sick from the stresses at work.

Stress relief is not the only benefit you may experience with constant practice of meditation. Meditation also has a profound effect on the mind and body by creating a balance that better prepares you to cope with challenging situations.

Meditation is simply exercised and requires little preparation or understanding. To benefit your overall physical and mental health, take some time out of your life for meditation and feel the power of a strong mind/body connection.

Stress in unavoidable in today's society and the better a person can manage it, the more a person will enjoy the many health benefits. To do this naturally greatly increases a person's wellbeing. Meditation is just one technique that can be used to manage your stress.

CLOSING

One of the most effective ways for managing stress could be as simple as relaxing and letting go of any tension in your body. You need to acknowledge the negative emotions and feelings, allowing them to come to the surface completely then letting go.

It's up to you to decide when you are ready to let go of this emotion. Once you have, simply relax any tension in the body, breathe, and let go.

Exhale deeply and imagine the negativity flowing out of your body to strengthen the effectiveness of the technique. It is a very simple stress management tool, but one that takes practice and persistence, it will not be a magic fix overnight. Don't give up.

The acknowledgment of your emotion is important. By fully recognizing and accepting how you are feeling and what might be causing the issues, you avoid running the risk of suppressing any negativity that may be driving you subconsciously. By bringing the negative feelings to the surface you are essentially taking the necessary steps to release it.

Deciding whether or not you're ready to let a particular emotion go is significant. This is because some emotions may be there to protect us from harm. Anger rather than passiveness, for instance, may be a more resourceful and useful state to be in if your safety - or even your life - is in danger.

A certain amount of aggression may be needed for you to push through and succeed at any kind of competitive sport - being in a more relaxed frame of mind in this situation may mean the difference between winning and losing.

Emotions therefore have their values and uses, and thus questioning yourself about whether you should and are ready to let go is a crucial step. Only you know whether you are ready to take that step.

This breathing and releasing method, once perfected, is a very powerful way of managing stress and the anxiety that can come with it. It can be repeated many, many times throughout the day, is fast, effective and discrete.

Over time you'll find it easier and easier to allow your body to relax and let go, and in turn you'll find it easier and easier to manage your stress and anxiety.

Best wishes. and breathe easy my friends.

-DSW

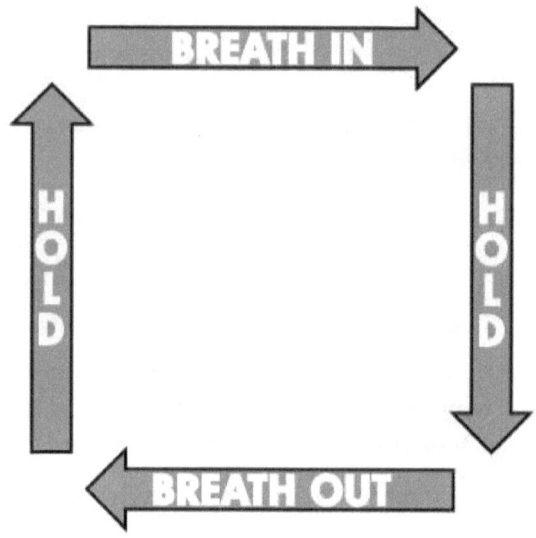

www.ingramcontent.com/pod-product-compliance
Lightning Source LLC
Chambersburg PA
CBHW031443210526
45464CB00005B/2318